Back
TO THE
Basics

The Book of Knowledge

ALIA WASH

Trans*formed*

Publishing

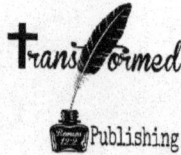

Mission: To Proclaim Transformation and Truth
Publisher: Transformed Publishing, Cocoa, FL
Website: www.transformedpublishing.com
Email: transformedpublishing@gmail.com

ISBN: 978-1-953241-50-4 (paperback)
ISBN: 978-1-953241-90-0 (hardcover)

Table of Contents

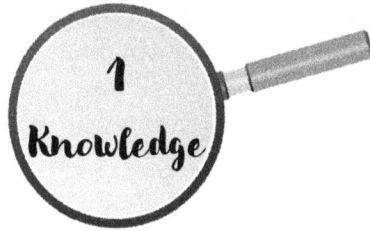

1

Knowledge

Knowledge (n.): the sum of what is known: the body of truth, information, and principles acquired by humankind[1]

This book was produced to open the eyes of God's people. It is a combination of things God has taught me over a three-year period in my personal pursuit to heal myself from lupus, fibromyalgia, diabetes, and mental illness. Through my journey, I have learned about my body, how it works, and what it needs to maintain my healing. God's desire is for our spiritual eyes to be open and allow the Holy Spirit that's on the inside of us to lead.

I am not a medical physician, but I am a self-taught herbalist as well as a homesteader who has healed myself. We are living in a day and time, now more than ever, when we have to get back to the basics of God - the way He intended us to be. He's been trying to get us back to the place we were with Him in the garden. Everything God made was good. The garden of Eden was made for man and woman, to tend and keep, as food for nourishment. God created fruits and vegetables. He set us up in the garden to be self-sufficient but through Him.

My prayer is that the Holy Spirit will speak to you as you read this book and empower you to see medicine as food, and food as medicine. I pray you will become more self-sufficient and live at your optimum health.

So, let's begin our journey together to acquire knowledge, wisdom, and understanding.

Blessings to you all!
Healing to you all who read this book!
Freedom to you all who read this book!
In Jesus name, let's begin . . .

My people are destroyed for lack of knowledge . . .
–Hosea 4:6

The only way to embark upon this work is to start at the beginning - during creation. After God made Adam and Eve, He set them in the Garden of Eden. They were made in His image. The setting He placed them in was the Garden of Eden, full of fruits and vegetables, beautiful vegetation, and all kinds of animals. He gave man rule over it all.

Every tree was pleasant for sight and good for food. In this garden, He put the man whom He had formed to dwell there and find fulfillment. Genesis 2:8-9 clearly demonstrates that God's intention was for us to receive sustenance and nourishment from the food He provided. It was pleasing to the eye and good for the body. There was one tree God commanded them *not* to partake of, called the tree of the knowledge of good and evil.

The Garden of Eden was pure and holy. It is my interpretation that God forbad them to eat of *this* tree because He had already provided them with all they needed. If they were to partake in the tree of the knowledge of good and evil, it would expose them to things He did not desire for them to encounter. Adam and Eve were in their purest form walking with Him in the cool of the day and always communing with Him because His spirit was there with them. They could rest assure in Him.

2
Deception

So when the woman saw that the tree *was* good for food, that it *was* pleasant to the eyes, and a tree desirable to make *one* wise, she took of its fruit and ate. She also gave to her husband with her, and he ate.

-Genesis 3:6

Deception came through a conversation with the serpent. The serpent deceived the woman who God had given man. It enticed her to know more and want more, even though she already had everything she needed. It is important to meditate on this point, as we go back down memory lane to the garden in the beginning.

Because of this act of disobedience to God, their eyes were opened, and they became aware they were uncovered – naked. Their immediate response was to hide from God. They thought He would no longer commune with them the way He did when He first placed them in the beautiful garden. I encourage you to read all of Genesis chapter 3 for yourself. God still desired fellowship with Adam and Eve. He talked to them about what happened, explained the consequences, made atonement - clothing them in tunics of skin, and evicted them from the garden so they wouldn't also partake of the tree of life, which would have left them permanently in a sinful state.

Now, outside the Garden of Eden, they were faced with the challenges of toiling instead of the productivity of tending. God truly intends for us to live and abide in prosperity here on this earth, as the healthiest and strongest versions of ourselves. God desires to draw us closer to Him than we have ever been before. Throughout this book, I pray He will open each reader's eyes to get back to Him.

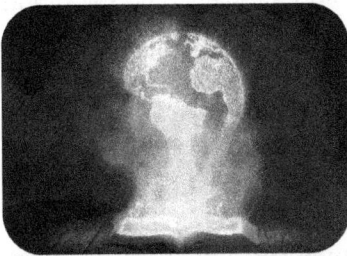

3
Our Bodies

Our Ten Body Systems

The only way to begin our journey is to identify and discuss God's original design of the human body. Over time, deception has shifted us away from the things God made for the nourishment of our bodies and from truly knowing our bodies, to know what makes it function, to know what keeps it healthy, and to know how it works.

A beautiful thing about the way God created the body is that it has its own filtration system. It has a *pumping system* to systematically cleanse and restore the body on its own. When the body is given what it needs, it is more apt to function correctly.

The human body consists of cells, tissues, and organs that work together to make life possible. It contains ten major systems, which are responsible for the body's functions: skeletal, muscular, cardiovascular, nervous, endocrine, lymphatic, respiratory, digestive, urinary, and reproductive.

The skeletal, muscular, cardiovascular, and nervous systems in particular create an infrastructure that facilitates the other systems. The adult **skeletal system** is a framework of over 200 bones holding the body together, giving it shape, and protecting its organs and tissues. The skeleton also provides anchor points for the **muscular system** which includes three types of muscles – skeletal, smooth, and cardiac. They are found throughout the body and facilitate movement. Nestled within these muscles is the **cardiovascular system**, a pipeline that includes the heart, blood vessels, and the blood itself. It is also called the circulatory system and delivers oxygen, white blood cells, hormones, and nutrients throughout the body. The **nervous system** is a communication network of nerve cells the body uses to transmit information and coordinate bodily functions. It's comprised of the brain (the hub of sensory and intellectual activity), the spinal cord, and the many cranial and spinal nerves that emanate from them. This infrastructure created by neurons, blood, muscles, and bones allows three other systems to regulate the body's environment: the endocrine, lymphatic, and urinary systems.

The **endocrine system** is a series of glands that use information carried by the nervous system to help regulate the body's processes. Thanks to this neural connection, endocrine glands, such as the thyroid, are aware of the number of hormones and other chemicals they need to produce. These chemicals are then distributed throughout the body, by way of the cardiovascular system.

The cardiovascular and nervous systems are also utilized by the **lymphatic system** (a collection of lymph nodes and vessels that help regulate the body's defenses). Also called the immune system, the lymphatic system uses neural pathways to transmit information about affected areas of the body and then sends out healing agents like white blood cells via the bloodstream.

Another key regulatory system is the **urinary system** which includes the kidneys, ureters, bladder, and urethra. The urinary or renal system maintains the body's electrolyte levels and filters waste from the blood. This waste is sent through the blood vessels, into the kidneys, and then expelled as urine.

All of these systems require energy to function. That's where the respiratory and digestive systems come in. The **respiratory system** is a group of passageways and organs that extract life giving oxygen from the air we breathe. Air enters the body through nasal cavities, travels down the throat, and is then transported to the lungs. The lungs extract oxygen for the body to use and then expel a carbon dioxide byproduct when we exhale.

Most energy comes in the form of food. The **digestive system** is an approximately 30-foot series of organs that convert food into fuel. Food enters the system through the mouth, then moves into the esophagus, and progresses through the stomach and intestines. The nutrients are absorbed into the body while solid waste is expelled through the anal canal which is the end of the digestive tract.

Humans are complicated organisms but when our ten major organ systems are healthy, they ensure our well-being. So now that we have gone through the body and we are more familiar with how all the systems work, let's dive into the five systems that help the body function at its optimum ability. It is important to be especially attentive to these systems.

Our Five Health Defense Systems[1]

BACK TO
THE BASICS
SUMMARY

Angiogenesis, which is how the body grows 60,000 miles worth of blood vessels.

Rejuvenation, the generation of our stem cells inside our bone marrow to circulate through our blood.

Microbiome, which has everything to do with our gut health.

DNA, our body's building blocks and protection from the environment.

Immune system, our body's defense mechanism. It's so powerful it can wipe out disease.

These systems are vital to maintaining a healthy body. You may be wondering, *Why should I know about these systems?* Well, our body is a machine so we should know all the working parts of it.

   ✓ How can I better take care of my body?
   ✓ What will help my body function properly?

Our body is like a car. Think about it. We must keep up with the maintenance of our car by checking the tires, oil, and other fluid levels that enable it to perform best. Most of us have experienced the stress and setback of a nail in the tire, low oil preventing the mechanical parts of the engine from seamlessly working together, or an overheating vehicle unable to take us to our destination. We know proper maintenance is key to maximizing the longevity of our vehicle. We must also know what it takes for our body to rejuvenate blood vessels, maintain proper gut health – microbiome, and things that affect our DNA and immune systems.

Angiogenesis is very important to the body because it generates new blood vessels throughout the body's lifespan. The body can rejuvenate new blood vessels daily if it has proper food and nutrition to be able to function at its highest capacity. Yes, our DNA can be rejuvenated as well and replenished daily. Our microbials are the key to all the working parts of the body because they process the food that fuels our body. Our immune system lives so it's essential to give our stomach and microbiome system what it needs to produce and maintain good gut bacteria, also known as probiotics, which can be found in foods, such as kiwi, sauerkraut, and kombucha, just to name a few.

Stem cells can rejuvenate also and aid in the regrowth of vital organs. For example, parts of the heart that are injured after a heart attack can be restored. Surprisingly, we're naturally regenerating every single day. Stem cells live in our bone marrow and organs. We've got more than seventy-five million of them, in our lungs, liver, skin, and even hidden in our fat. They help our body regenerate daily. You may be wondering, *Where is the proof?* Think about it, our hair grows back, our skin grows back, and the lining of our gut sloughs off and grows back. Did you know that if the tip of the lung is removed or has been injured by a disease such as COVID or pneumonia, it can grow back? This is also true for the liver! Even if two thirds of a liver is removed, and only one third of it is left, just with that little nub, the entire liver can grow back! Saying our bodies are amazing is an understatement!

Did you know dark chocolate can aid in the release and production of new stem cells from your own bone marrow? Yes, eating dark bitter chocolate can help our body repair itself.

God perfectly created each interrelated system in our body and caused the earth to bring forth what is needed to nourish it and keep it well so we can live a quality life! In His infinite wisdom, God made our human body able to heal thyself.

As it is commonly said, "Knowing is half the battle." Maybe you are like me before I embarked on this journey to learn how to heal myself from lupus, fibromyalgia, and diabetes. I did not have knowledge of any of the information I am now sharing. I never partnered with my doctor. I just trusted him or her to tell me what was wrong and how to fix it. When I began to empower myself by taking seminars, reading books, studying *my* body and what it took to make it heal itself, I began to think about how amazing God really is. He gave us everything we need from the very beginning, so why do we trust everything else but God?

The information I previously shared about the Five Health Defense Systems, I learned from a master class I participated in taught by Dr. William Li. He is a physician, scientist, professor, and author of the book, *Eat to Beat Disease*.

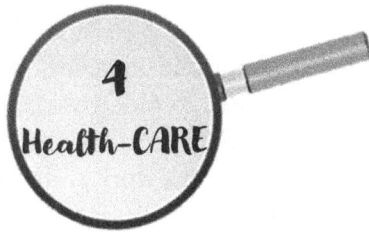

4

Health-CARE

Now let's dive into what it takes to keep these five health systems in our body working properly and make them work for us.

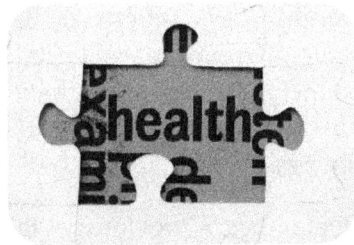

We must restart and rewire our body from poor eating habits and damage to our DNA through exposure to contaminates we unknowingly breathe, encounter, or ingest from the microwave we use, to the chemicals in our food because of the pesticides used on crops or antibiotics given to the livestock we consume.

Cleansing the Body

I discovered that if I wanted to purge my body of lupus, fibromyalgia, and diabetes, I must first do a cleanse to eliminate my body of toxins, impurities, undigested meat, and processed foods lingering in my gut and contributing to my sickness. We must determine the best type of fasting for our desired outcome, learn *how* to start and finish a successful fast, and *do* it.

Fasting:

> But as for me, when they were sick,
> My clothing was sackcloth;
> I humbled myself with fasting;
> And my prayer would return to my own heart.
> —Psalm 35:13

13

Fasting is a way to humble ourselves in the sight of God. Not only can we get closer to God by fasting, but we reboot all our health systems. The digestive system shuts down because it doesn't have to work so hard to break down food and allows our body to focus on other things. Fasting has been associated with several health benefits including weight loss, improved blood sugar control, decreased inflammation, and enhanced heart health. So, not only do we connect in a deeper more intimate way with God spiritually, but we also jump start the healing process within our physical body.

Remember, I previously stated, we are to *partner* with our doctor(s), so it is important to consult with your trusted medical professional regarding the appropriate fast for you. Throughout this book, I am speaking from my personal research and experience. My words are not meant to condemn anyone or override medical recommendations. There are different types of fasts. I used water fasting to begin my healing process and know it was and *is* pivotal to my healing journey.

Water Fasting:

Our body is made up of fifty to seventy-five percent water.[1] Every organ and system uses water to get rid of toxins and regulate itself correctly. Water fasting activates metabolism, improves the skin, cleanses cells, and aids brain function. Water fasting also *kicks* our body into **ketosis,** usually on the third day of fasting.

> **Ketosis** is a process that happens when your body doesn't have enough carbohydrates to burn for energy. Instead, it burns fat and makes things called ketones, which it can use for fuel.[2]

Research has shown ketosis may have several health benefits including weight loss. Eating less food can help decrease belly fat while maintaining a lean mass. During the ketosis process, old cells die, and new cells regenerate. Fasting is imperative because it *kick starts* the benefits of rejuvenation, one of the five health systems.

Other types of fasts you may decide to embark upon are summarized below:

Liquid Fast:

Only consume liquids (water, fruit / vegetable juice, and / or broth).

The Daniel Fast:

This is a Biblical fast, usually a twenty-one-day duration to eliminate meats and other animal products, sweets, breads, and preservatives from our diet. Drink water and juice. Eat fruits, vegetables, and other foods from the ground such as whole grains, nuts, and seeds (raw, juiced, or cooked). The Daniel Fast benefits the body by promoting healthy skin, healthy digestion, healthy hormonal balance, improving energy, breaking sugar addiction, and connecting us closer to God.

Intermittent Fasting:

Not eating food for consecutive hours during the day.

Additional Benefits of Fasting:

Fasting will usually result in weight loss, reduced body fat, reduced levels of perceived stress, increased ketogenesis, decreased blood sugar levels, lower risk of some diseases, and initiate **autophagy**.

Autophagy is your body's process of reusing old and damaged cell parts. Cells are the basic building blocks of every tissue and organ in your body. Each cell contains multiple parts that keep it functioning. Over time, these parts can become defective or stop working. They become litter, or junk, inside an otherwise healthy cell.

Autophagy is your body's cellular recycling system. It allows a cell to disassemble its junk parts and repurpose the salvageable bits and pieces into new, usable cell parts. A cell can discard the parts it doesn't need.

Autophagy is also quality control for your cells. Too many junk components in a cell take up space and can slow or prevent a cell from functioning correctly. Autophagy remakes the clutter into the selected cell components you need, optimizing your cells' performance.[3]

5
Cell-CARE

Most recent estimates put the number of cells at around 30 trillion. Written out, that's 30,000,000,000,000! These cells all work in harmony to carry out all the basic functions necessary for humans to survive.[1]

Each cell has to eat, poop (eliminate waste), move, migrate, and produce its designated assignment. Cells breathe and release carbon dioxide. When the body is in a more acidic state, it is more conducive for cancerous cells because the cellular rejuvenation process becomes hindered. There are ways to keep our body from forming **acidosis,** a condition in which there is too much acid in the body fluids[2], resulting in constipation of cells and depletion of structural function. We must cleanse our lymphatic system by eating ample fruits and vegetables which flush out the lymph nodes. Applying ginger oil while massaging our lymph nodes pushes toxins from the body and promotes cell rejuvenation and proper function.

> The **lymphatic system** is a circulatory system made up of lymph vessels, which are much like blood vessels. It drains extra fluid (called lymph) that has passed out of the blood and into tissues and returns it back to the blood. The lymphatic system also includes tissues and organs that make, store and release lymphocytes (a type of white blood cell).
>
> These tissues and organs (called lymphatic or lymphoid tissue) also monitor the lymph for germs,

foreign substances and abnormal cells and remove waste products and bacteria from the lymph.

The lymphatic system includes the tonsils, spleen, thymus, lymph nodes and lymph vessels and is an important part of the immune system that helps defend the body against disease. It also helps maintain blood pressure and transports some hormones, nutrients and waste products.[3]

The Lymphatic System

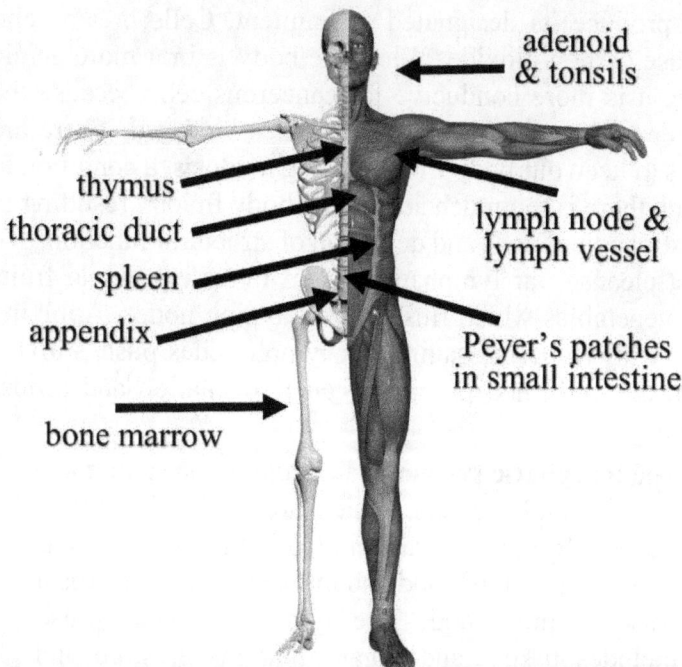

adenoid & tonsils

thymus

thoracic duct

spleen

appendix

bone marrow

lymph node & lymph vessel

Peyer's patches in small intestine

The lymphatic system is important for the optimum functioning of our general and specific immune responses. The lymph nodes monitor the lymph flowing into them and produce cells and antibodies which protect our body from infection and disease. Seasonal cleansing of the body is essential. Let us care for the body that cares for us!

Lymphatic Cleanse

It is very important to the health systems that the lymph nodes work properly. Lymph nodes are designed to cleanse the body of infection and even cancer cells. If they aren't working properly, it could affect the entire immune system. It is imperative to *help* the lymphatic system out. This can be accomplished by drinking plenty of water, walking, and giving yourself a lymphatic massage. Heavens Cure Natural Foods offers ginger oil which is amazing for cleansing the lymph nodes and reduces inflammation.

Please scan the QR Code to watch a video from my YouTube channel demonstrating, *How to do a lymphatic massage using my ginger oil.*

6
My Journey

As I began the cleansing process in my body, I went on a fourteen day fast. I ate nothing and only drank distilled water, alkaline water, and spring water. The first couple of days I was hungry, I had a headache, and it was hard to sleep. After my body went into ketosis it started to use and burn stored fat and demolish the badly diseased cells that were in my body. Throughout the duration of my fourteen day fast, I did not take my medication. This was my own personal decision, and I am not advising anyone to *not* take their medication. I decided to eliminate everything from my body, including the medication. It was a risk I was willing to take, *anything* and *everything*, to be free of the diseases that were infiltrating my body.

One of the most important things to remember about going on a journey of healing and obtaining the knowledge you need to do so, is that you must have a *made-up mind*, sold out and ready to *do* something different to transition to a different lifestyle and a different way of thinking about food. It is imperative to reprogram your mind, body, and spirit to know, *You can do it!* What do you have to lose? I was tired of taking so many medications, tired of the pain, and most of all tired of not having the quality of life I knew I deserved. I had the realization that disease was a state of mind, and I chose to live.

Now, just because I started my journey the way I did doesn't mean you have to follow my exact path, but I do encourage you to find and follow the path that is right for you.

7
Parasites

I am thankful for all the knowledge I obtained while researching different fasting methods. I also discovered important facts to really enhance my healing journey as it pertains to cleansing the body. Cleansing should begin with a deep parasite cleanse. The reason being parasites extract the nutrients from our body. They can be hidden in different places, such as our muscles, brain, intestines, pancreas, and / or spleen. These parasites can be the leading cause of disease plaguing our body.

Parasitism is a close relationship between species, where one organism, the parasite, lives on or inside another organism, the host, causing it some harm, and is adapted structurally to this way of life. The entomologist E. O. Wilson characterized parasites as "predators that eat prey in units of less than one".[1]

What does a parasite infestation do to the human body?

These invaders can wreak havoc on your entire body, from your brain to your liver. Some of them have the potential to cause problems that can last years. Parasites can also contribute to inflammation, immune impairment, and even autoimmune activation.[2]

This is why it is so important to eliminate the parasites from our body prior to cleansing the disease the parasites carry and infiltrate in our body.

How do humans contract parasites?

Anyone can contract a parasitic infection and some people are at higher risk. Infestation can happen from touching objects or surfaces with parasite eggs on them that enter the body or ingesting contaminated water or food. Awareness, cleanliness, and good personal hygiene limit the spread of parasites.

One of the most common ways to contract parasites through food is by eating undercooked meat. Different types of parasites can plague the human body. Protozoa, helminths, and ectoparasites are the three main classes of parasites that can cause disease in humans.

A common helminth infests humans known as the pinworm, seatworm, nematode, or roundworm.

> It is the most prevalent nematode in the United States. Humans are the only known host, and about 209 million persons worldwide are infected. More than 30 percent of children worldwide are infected.[3]

This is why it's so important to start with a parasite cleanse.

How should I prepare my body for a parasite cleanse?

As we embark upon our health journey, it is important to begin to eat *clean*. To eat clean is to cut all starches from the diet, including eliminating all pasta, bread, and sugar. It is impossible to do a successful cleanse, and still consume processed sugar and starch. Parasites feed on sugars and starches. Also eliminate dairy from your diet. Animal milk is not meant for the human body to consume, so that is why it's on this list of things that should not be consumed while preparing for a cleansing.

Preparation is key when cleansing the body. Cut back, then remove these items from your diet to begin to shut down the digestive system. Entering this process spontaneously will bring about the different side effects that come from doing it all at once. Parasitic cleansing is pivotal to a successful renewal and rejuvenation of the body.

Consume fruits and vegetables, raw or juiced, it is really up to you. Decrease meals to one a day to gradually wean the body from food. For the best results, dedicate seven days to prepare the body for the cleanse. Remember to always stay hydrated. Drink plenty of spring water, alkaline water, and coconut water. The next step is to begin your parasite cleanse.

How can I naturally eliminate parasites from my body?

Below is a list of various items that will naturally eliminate parasites. Select the ones that are right for you and follow the recommended serving sizes on the label.

Walnut Hull: (worm and parasite eliminator)
Black walnut hull is a viable herb that eliminates illnesses caused by ringworms, pinworms, tapeworms, and many other parasites. Walnut hull is a laxative, antiseptic, germicide, and a parasite eliminator.

Wormwood: (induced worm paralysis, death and ultrastructural alternations)[4]

Wormwood is used for various digestion problems such as loss of appetite, upset stomach, gall bladder disease, and intestinal spasms. Wormwood is also used to treat fever, liver disease, and worm infections; to increase sexual desire; as a tonic; and to stimulate sweating.[5]

Clove: (powerful anthelmintic, antiparasitic)
Clove is a vermifuge, or worm killing herb. It kills parasites and heals the stomach from the waste extracted from the death of the parasites.

Papaya Seeds: (help boost the immune system by removing toxins from the body)
Papaya seeds can be used as one of the keys to a parasite free gut. The seeds are used to flush parasites from the intestines. They can be blended into your smoothies.

Eucalyptus Oil: (strengthens the skin's natural barrier)
Eucalyptus oil contains antimicrobial properties to fight pathogens.

All these steps can be used to promote a successful deep parasitical cleanse which is the starting point to rejuvenate the cells that were destroyed through bad eating habits, as well as exposure to the elements of this world.

8
Nutrition

Healing yourself is a journey that requires lifestyle dietary changes. By learning *your* body, the purpose and steps to cleansing it, eliminating parasites, and resetting the body, you are well on your way to becoming a better version of yourself. Remember, the desire *to be a better version of ourselves* is not comparative, competitive, nor impossible to obtain. We are not aiming to *be* someone else.

Working knowledge of the body, the health systems, the rejuvenation process, and the body's ability to reverse disease, should propel and motivate us to maximize the body's productivity by eating healthy. In this chapter we will dive into a variety of foods that can lead us to our optimum health.

Throughout my personal pursuit of healing and learning how to maintain a healthy lifestyle, I acquired several books and applied the knowledge I gleaned from each author. I highly recommend for you also to passionately seek solutions and yield to God's direction. Being immersed in problems, quickly wearies our strength, therefore we must seek, find, and practice hopeful positive alternatives. I will share some excerpts that continue to impact and propel my mindset. Each has helped me to achieve outcomes, exceeding my original goals, when I started my journey.

Dr. William Li empathizes in his masterclass and book titled, *Eat to Beat Disease*, that food and nutrition are paramount to our health.

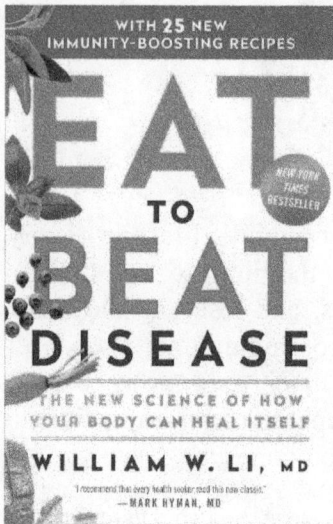

Sustainability goals requirement: by 2050, global consumption of fruits and vegetables, nuts, and legumes will have to double, and consumption of foods such as red meat, and sugar will have to be reduced by more than 50 percent.

Meaning, we must be intentional about adding more fruits and vegetables to our diet and removing sugars and meats to successfully beat disease and reap the benefits of self-sustainable health.

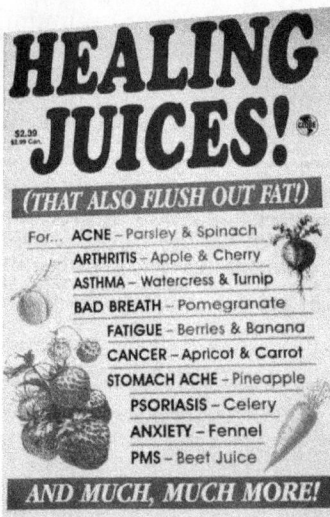

A book I go back to again and again is *Healing Juices* by L. A. Justice. It shares the benefits of a variety of fruits, vegetables, and nuts.

L. A. Justice emphasizes the advantages of juicing and provides easy-to-follow recipes we can make in our own homes. The cover is a preview of the great deal of knowledge shared in this book. Here is a sneak peak of the types of recipes you will find in *Healing Juices,* by L.A. Justice.

Anti-Allergy Juice (yields 3 cups)

Ingredients:
1 Cucumber, peeled
2 Stalks of Celery
1 Bunch of Spinach
1/2 Head of Broccoli
1 Pinch of Parsley
1/2 Cup of Ice (or bottled water to thin)

Directions:
Blend All

Cleansing Cocktail (yields 1 cup)

Ingredients:
2 Apples
1 Pear
1 Teaspoon of Lemon Juice
1 Small Piece of Ginger

Directions:
Blend All
Drink Daily (or every other day to stay regular)

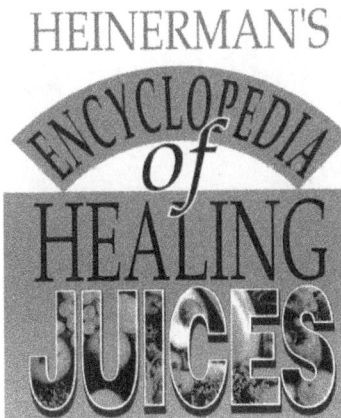

John Heinerman contrasts eating and juicing fruits and vegetables in his book *Encyclopedia of Healing Juices:*

Juicing works, so why not eat produce? Why not enjoy the sweet crunch of an apple or the soft smooth texture of a banana? The answer is simple: because it takes much longer to

HEINERMAN'S
ENCYCLOPEDIA
of
HEALING
JUICES

JOHN HEINERMAN
Foreword by Dr. Lendon Smith

From a medical anthropologist's files, here are Nature's own
healing juices for hundreds of today's most common health problems

digest whole fruits and vegetables. Juices are quickly and efficiently absorbed by the body-sometimes within minutes of consumption. For example, celery is well known as an effective antidote for the effects of heat exhaustion because of its high sodium chloride content but it would take hours to find relief by actually eating a few stalks. Drinking a glass of celery juice, however, brings very quick relief from the symptoms. But you can't just chug it. Instead, you should sip the juice slowly through a straw. By doing so, the tongue has the added benefit of having the juice run over its taste buds and linger a little while before being swallowed.

Please scan the QR Code to watch a video from my YouTube channel demonstrating juicing, *Pure Hydration, Come On and Juice with Me.*

Most foods can be classified as alkaline or acidic. It is important for our body that we consume more alkaline foods.

Shayna Komar, RD, LD, a licensed and registered dietitian at Cancer Wellness, weighs in on the debate.

Some background: The alkaline diet is based around the idea that the foods you eat can alter the acidity or alkalinity (the pH value) of your body, explains Komar. On a scale of 0 to 14, a pH of 0 to 6 is considered acidic, while a pH of 7 to 14 is considered alkaline.

"There is some early evidence that eating a more alkaline food plan can help with weight loss, prevent kidney stones, keep bones and muscles strong, improve cardiovascular health and brain function, and reduce the risk of type 2 diabetes," she says.[1]

The more acidic the body is, the more disease the body accumulates. The more alkaline the body is, the healthier and stronger the body will be. Studies continue to support that our body's optimum health is achieved from maintaining an alkaline pH level and that level is affected by the foods we eat.

Life on earth depends on appropriate pH levels in and around living organisms and cells. Human life requires a tightly controlled pH level in the serum of about 7.4 (a slightly alkaline range of 7.35 to 7.45) to survive.[2]

I have included a list of alkaline foods on the next page. This is not all inclusive list.

Alkaline Foods List
*This is not an all inclusive list.

Vegetables
Amaranth Greens
Avocado
Dandelion Greens
Green Banana
Kale
Lettuce (not iceberg)
Mushroom
(not shitake)
Mexican Cactus
Nopales
Okra
Olives
Onions
Peppers
Purslane
Sea Vegetables
(nori, dulse, kelp,
sea moss, etc.)
Squash
Tomatillos
Tomatoes
(plum & cherry)
Turnip Greens
Watercress Greens
Zucchini
Wild Arugula

Nuts, Beans, & Seeds
Almonds
Brazilian Nuts
Chestnuts
Coconut
Flax Seeds
Hemp Seeds
Pumpkin Seeds
Sesame Seeds
Sunflower Seeds
Walnuts

Butters
Tahini
Walnut

Fruits
Apples
Burro Banana
Berries
(no cranberries)
Cactus Fruit
Cherries
Currants
Dates
Figs
Grapes w/ seeds
Key Limes
Mangos
Melons
Oranges
Papaya
Peaches
Pears
Plums
Raisins
Soft Jelly Coconuts
Soursop
Tamarind

Seasonings
Achiote
Agave
Basil
Bay Leaf
Cayenne Pepper
Date Sugar
Dill
Habanero
Onion Powder
Oregano
Sage
Savory
Sea Salt
Tarragon
Thyme

Oils
Avocado / Coconut
Flax / Grapeseed
Olive / Sesame

Grains
Amaranth
Fonio
Kamut
Millet
Quinoa
Rye
Teff
Wild Rice

Beans & Legumes
Chickpeas
Lima
Mung
Navy
Pinto
Red
Soy
White

Sprouts
Alfalfa
Amaranth
Broccoli
Fenugreek
Kamut
Mung Bean
Quinoa
Radish
Soy
Spelt

Flour
Almond
Coconut
Cassava
Tigernut
Green Banana
Chestnut
& Arrowroot

We've learned a lot about our body and our health systems. We also now know how to cleanse our body through different types of fasting, eliminate parasites, and eat to maintain our body in an alkaline state to beat disease. This information supports the statement, *food is medicine*. In the next chapter, we will learn additional natural ways to assist the body to heal by using natural medicine. Let's dive into herbal medicine.

9
Natural Medicine

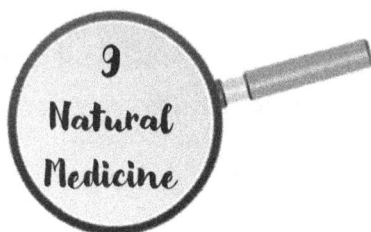

Herbal supplements have helped me to maintain my healing. My personal life experiences and the research I continue to do, support my belief that God intended for the body to combat disease *naturally*.

Disclaimer:

Please be advised, I am not a doctor. I am a self-taught herbalist who healed myself by being obedient to the Holy Spirit's prompting. Now, I share what helped me because I am confident my story and research can also help others. Please collaborate with God and your doctor before using any natural herbal supplements.

Now Let's Begin:

Herbal supplements are plant based. Many plants grown naturally from the earth have medicinal properties that can be used to regulate and eliminate high blood pressure, diabetes, heart disease, liver issues, blood disorders, and circulation problems; reduce stress; reverse infertility; improve stamina; and treat an array of other health issues.

In this chapter, I am sharing the benefits of many herbal supplements that are readily available. They are listed in alphabetical order. The supplements marked with an asterisk (*), are available through my online store, *Heavens Cure Natural Foods.*

https://heavenscurenaturalfoods.com/

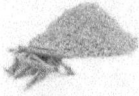

*Ashwaganda Root

Reduces anxiety and stress. Fights depression. Boosts fertility, testosterone in men, and brain function.

*Astragalus

Used in ancient Chinese medicine. It is great for lymphatic detox and is an anti-inflammatory, antifungal, and antiparasitic. Astragalus is known to protect blood vessels and lower cholesterol.

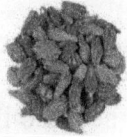

*Black Cardamom Pods

This nut is used to lower blood pressure and protect from chronic diseases. It acts as an anti-inflammatory, helps alleviate digestive problems including ulcers, treats bad breath, prevents cavities, has an antibacterial effect, provides respiratory relief, and contains cancer fighting compounds. Available in pods, powder, & capsules.

*Bladderwrack

Protects your gut (gastrointestinal tract). Relieves diarrhea and constipation. Soothes the stomach. Lubricates and repairs intestinal walls. Improves bowel movements. Noted to have anti-obesity, anti-inflammatory, antioxidant, and anti-carcinogenic benefits.

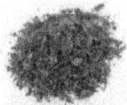

*Borage

This plant's flowers and leaves can be used to treat fevers and coughs. It is also an option to alleviate depression and is used for a hormone problem called adrenal insufficiency, for blood purification, to increase urine flow, to prevent inflammation of the lungs, as a sedative, and to promote sweating.

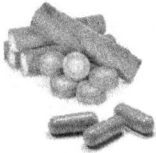

*Burdock Root

Full of medicinal qualities especially ones for lymph detox. It's a great detoxifier, as a diuretic it flushes toxins out of the body.

Offers therapeutic benefits in the case of high blood pressure, gout, hepatitis and other liver diseases. It also helps regulate blood sugar levels.

For your lymph detox, include burdock root to relieve any spleen and tonsil swelling or infection. In other words, burdock root recharges our lymph organs.

Calendula

The leaves of this are used in tinctures and ointments to wash and treat burns, bruises, and cuts. It also helps to eliminate infections, prevents dermatitis or skin inflammation, and is used by people with breast cancer during radiation therapy.

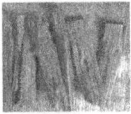

*Cat's Claw

This bark is known to treat HIV, HPV, herpes, Alzheimer's, arthritis, diverticulitis, peptic ulcers, colitis, gastritis, hemorrhoids, parasites, and leaky bowel syndrome. It also fights against cancer.

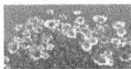

*Chamomile

This plant contains anti-inflammatory properties. It soothes cold symptoms, is good for the heart, helps with digestion and sleep, reduces anxiety, soothes sore throat, and supports the immune system.

Chaparral

A botanical extract claimed to have beneficial effects for many conditions from skin rashes to cancer to herpes to snake bites. It can also be used for pain and inflammation, diabetes, digestive problems, and it can treat gallbladder issues and kidney stones.

*Chicory Root Powder

Used to regulate appetite, ease upset stomach, relieve constipation, and treat liver and gallbladder disorders, cancer, and rapid heartbeat.

*Dandelion

Dandelion acts as a diuretic, increasing the amount of urine the body makes. The leaves are used to stimulate the appetite and help digestion. The flower is an antioxidant. The root can be used to strengthen the heart to fight against heart disease.

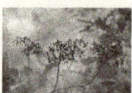

*Elderberry

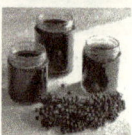

Derives from the elderberry tree. The berries are used as medicine. It can be made into teas or tinctures. Elderberry boosts the immune system, helps tame inflammation, lessens stress, helps protect the heart and is packed with antioxidants to help ease cold, flu, and allergy symptoms.

Fenugreek

This plant is beneficial in lowering blood sugar, boosting testosterone, and increasing milk production in breast-feeding women. It also helps to reduce belly fat and contains compounds that are good for hair growth.

*Flaxseed

This seed is used to improve digestive health, relieve constipation, reduce the risk of heart disease, lower cholesterol, and fight against belly fat.

*Frankincense Resin

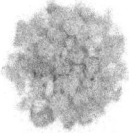

This resin is used to treat tumors, toothaches, arthritis, cold, cough, and various inflammatory conditions.

*Ginger Root Powder

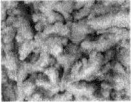

An anti-inflammatory helps ease nausea, reduces blood pressure, relieves headaches and migraines, and is a rich antioxidant. Available as a powder, drink, and oil.

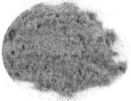

Gotu Kola

This plant is used to treat varicose veins and chronic venous insufficiency. It fights against conditions where the blood pools in the leg. Also, used as an ointment to treat psoriasis and helps heal minor wounds. Beneficial when treating Alzheimer's, reduces anxiety and stress, and is used as an antidepressant.

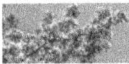

Hawthorne

Hawthorne is used to help protect against heart disease, control high blood pressure and high cholesterol, it increases coronary artery blood flow and improves circulation.

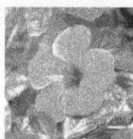

*Hibiscus

The hibiscus plant is rich in antioxidants such as beta-carotene, vitamin C, and much more. It fights inflammation, lowers blood pressure, lowers cholesterol, promotes weight loss, fights bacteria, and supports liver health.

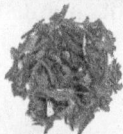

*Horsetail Tea

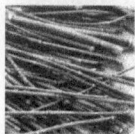

This plant is used to relieve fluid retention, kidney and bladder stones, urinary tract infections, as well as other contentious and general disturbances of the kidney and bladder.

Lemon Balm

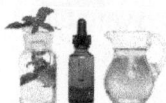

A member of the mint family, this plant is used to reduce stress and anxiety, promotes sleep, improves appetite, and ease pain and discomfort caused by digestion problems (bloating, gas, and colitis).

*Lion's Mane Powder

Derived from a mushroom. It contains compounds that may stimulate growth of new brain cells, improve depression and anxiety, and support heart and immune health.

*Lungwort

Used for breathing conditions, stomach and intestinal ailments, and kidney and urinary tract problems. Lungwort relieves fluid retention and treats lung disease and tuberculosis.

*Maca Root Powder

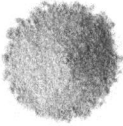

This adaptogen plant gives our body the ability to adapt or resist what's going on in and around it, including anxiety and depression. It also increases energy.

Marshmallow Leaf and Root

Used for pain and swelling, as well as inflammation of the mucous membranes that line the respiratory tract, dry cough, inflammation of the lining of the stomach, diarrhea, stomach ulcers, constipation, urinary tract infections, and stones in the urinary tract.

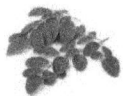

*Moringa

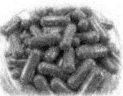

Taken by mouth and helps alleviate arthritis and other joint pain, asthma, cancer, constipation, diabetes, diarrhea, seizures, stomach pain, intestinal ulcers, intestinal spasms, headaches, heart problems, high blood pressure, kidney stones, symptoms of menopause, and thyroid disorder. When applied directly to the skin, it helps treat infections. Can be used as a germ killer or drying agent, and even reduces abscesses.

Motherwort

An anti-inflammatory with antioxidant effects, fights against bacteria, and stimulates the uterus. Motherwort can also help to prevent and stop excess bleeding.

Nettle

Stinging nettle has been used for hundreds of years to treat muscle and joint pain, eczema, arthritis, gout, anemia, and urinary tract infections. Promotes hair growth and cleanses the blood.

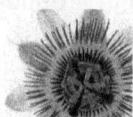

*Passionflower

This plant is known to reduce anxiety, help with sleep difficulties, pain, heart rhythm problems, menopause symptoms, and attention deficit hyperactive disorder.

Rosehip

A part of the rose flower that may boost the immune system, aid weight loss, reduce joint pain, support healthy looking skin, and protect against heart disease and type 2 diabetes.

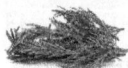

*Rosemary

This plant is used to alleviate muscle pain, improve memory, boost the immune and circulatory systems, and promote hair growth.

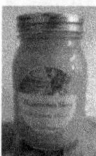

*Sea Moss

Sea moss is an alga, native to warmer ocean waters. It is packed with powerful minerals, containing 92 of the 102 minerals our body is made of. It is good for heart health, promotes healthy weight loss, and is a good source of iodine. Supports gut health, boosts the immune system, builds muscle mass, aids recovery after workouts, and helps to lower A1C levels. Overall, it is an essential natural supplement for the human body.

Skullcap

Known as a significant antioxidant, helps to protect against neurological disorders, such as Alzheimer's and Parkinson's disease, along with anxiety and depression.

St. John's Wort

This plant is used to help treat depression, menopausal symptoms, hyperactivity disorder (ADHD), somatic symptoms of extreme irritation and anxiety, and obsessive-compulsive disorder and conditions. It is also used as an antidiuretic.

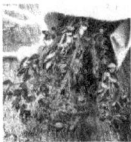

Thyme

Used for bacterial and fungal infections. Relieves coughing. Has an antioxidant effect. Slows hair loss conditions, such as alopecia. Listed as a plant to help treat dementia and many other conditions.

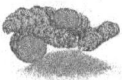

*Turmeric Root Powder

Known to treat pain, inflammation, hay fever, depression, high cholesterol, liver disease, itchiness, and osteoarthritis. Warning, this has a blood thinning property, do not take with other blood thinners. Available as a powder, drink, and tincture.

Valerian Root

The root of this flowering plant has medicinal purposes. It is used for insomnia, anxiety, depression, premenstrual syndrome (PMS), menopause symptoms, and headaches. It is known to be good for people who are fighting against schizophrenia.

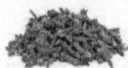 ## *Whole Cloves*

Improves respiratory conditions, provides relief from toothaches, improves digestion, acts as a natural refresher, treats nausea and vomiting, provides relief from inflammation and pain, helps control blood sugar levels, improves liver health, and eliminates parasites from the body.

Summary:

These are *some* of the herbs that can help us maintain our body's healing. However, these are just to name a few. There are many plants beholding powerful benefits we can consume with less detrimental effects on the body than synthetic medications.

There are so many side effects and other problems that can be caused by using synthetic medications. That was the number one reason I chose to go on this journey. After taking over fifteen pills a day for fifteen years, I developed other ailments related to synthetic medications. I knew deep down inside that my body was rejecting it and I was getting sicker and sicker. Through my studies and my results, I have found a new way of life.

Different seasons bring forth different herbs which can be consumed as teas, powders, or capsules. In the book titled, *Radical Remedies: An Herbalist Guide to Empowered Self Care*, the author Brittany Duncan shares herbs for each season:

Winter

ashwagandha, damiana, elderberry, ginger, lemon balm, licorice, nettle, oats, rosemary, St John's wort

Spring

burdock root, chamomile, chickweed, dandelion leaf, gotu kola, nettle, violet

Summer

calendula, hawthorne, hibiscus, marshmallow root, motherwort, passionflower, rose hip, skullcap

Autumn

elecampane, ginger, holy basil / tulsi, rose hip, thyme

All these plants are good for medicine and can help to maintain optimum health. The wealth of information I shared are suggestive measures to help others who may be looking to heal themselves from the ailments they battle with, as I personally did from lupus, fibromyalgia, diabetes, and mental illness.

Herbal remedies can also help with PTSD, bipolar / manic disorder, schizophrenia, anxiety, and sleep deprivation.

Other Remedies

Castor Oil

Derived from the castor seed, this oil is one of the deepest penetrating healing oils pressed for the body. It is widely known to eliminate constipation and can heal bone spurs. Apply it to a cloth and wrap the area for six to eight hours and repeat. It can be used to cleanse the liver by placing a saturated castor oil cloth under the right rib and binding it around the waist. Castor oil is also able to shrink fibroids as well as tumors with the same method as above. For the best results, incorporate a heating pad for extra activation.

*Microgreens

May improve heart health, fights against and helps treat Alzheimer's disease and cancer. Microgreens are a great source of vitamins (A, E, C, & K) and minerals such as calcium, magnesium, iron, selenium, and zinc. Nutritionally dense, which means you can receive the minerals and vitamins from the plant at a more accelerated rate.

Homegrown microgreens are a safer and healthier way to go for optimum health. Generally, foods manufactured in laboratories are contaminated with added chemicals, which can negatively impact our health in many ways. Grow your own food or purchase homegrown foods from local farmers. Good news, *Heavens Cure Natural Foods*, also has microgreens available.

*Turmeric Ginger Bomb (recipe on next page!)

Useful for many different ailments. Helps relieve pain, indigestion, fever, nausea, and inflammation.

Garlic & Honey Fermented (recipe on next page!)

Known to be great for the immune system, has antibacterial and antiviral properties that can help ward off disease, and is a natural antibiotic.

Hydration

True hydration isn't obtained by drinking water alone. It is actually possible to drink too much water. Excessive water intake not only flushes the cells but can throw off your salt and potassium ratio. This causes the body to retain too much water. H3O2 is a natural electrolyte. It is found in coconut water, cucumbers, and watermelon, to name a few. Drink your fruits!

Turmeric Ginger Bomb

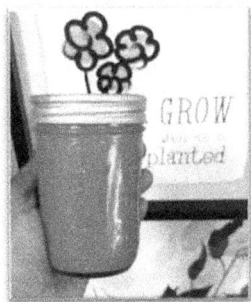

Ingredients:
1 cup of turmeric
1/2 cup of ginger
1/2 teaspoon of cayenne pepper or black pepper
honey (to taste)

Directions:
Mix all ingredients in a mason jar
Add honey
Stir until it is completely blended (like a paste)

Use:
The paste can be used in teaspoon portions orally (in tea, coffee, water, to cook with, or taken alone)

Garlic & Honey Fermented

Ingredients:
1 cup of raw garlic (sliced)
Raw honey

Directions:
Fill mason jar with raw garlic
Completely immerse the garlic in raw honey
Place the sealed mason jar into a dark area for 24 hours or until the honey has become liquefied

10
Choices

It is my prayer that through my studies, I can pass on this book of knowledge, to catapult others into a new lifestyle of healing oneself. It has been through the help of God, our Creator, who created *all* plants and us, and the inspiration of the Holy Spirit, that I was even able to heal myself. It started from one simple thought, *Alia, you can do this!*

Changing the way I viewed food was an essential key to the self-healing transformation that took place in my mind, body, and spirit. Most importantly, I genuinely desire each day to become a better version of myself. By sharing my story, I hope to encourage you to also crave the healthier and stronger version of yourself, resulting in you becoming more self-sufficient.

There are so many processed foods being introduced into our society that have discreetly become part of our diet. Such contaminants as high fructose corn syrup change our body's natural way of processing sugar, causing different diseases, and producing excess mucus in the body. These factors promote sickness which in turn makes us dependent upon man-made synthetic medications. *So, why process foods?* To manufacture food at a faster rate.

Where does high fructose corn syrup (HFCS) come from?

HFCS is derived from corn starch. Starch itself is a chain of glucose (a simple sugar) molecules joined together.

When corn starch is broken down into individual glucose molecules, the end product is corn syrup, which is essentially 100% glucose.

To make HFCS, enzymes are added to corn syrup in order to convert some of the glucose to another simple sugar called fructose, also called "fruit sugar" because it occurs naturally in fruits and berries.

HFCS is 'high' in fructose compared to the pure glucose that is in corn syrup. Different formulations of HFCS contain different amounts of fructose.[1]

What are the side effects of consuming high fructose corn syrup?

Ingestion of fructose chronically has contributed to multiple health consequences, such as insulin resistance, obesity, liver disorders, and diabetes. Studies have shown excessive consumption of high fructose corn syrup can be toxic to the liver. It is also considered a primary cause of obesity in America.

Weight gain abetted by high-calorie foods containing HFCS can also contribute to heart disease, diabetes, fatty liver disease and dyslipidemia, an abnormal level of cholesterol and other fats in the blood. Fructose becomes a more universal threat to your body by accumulating as visceral fat around your organs.[2]

What foods contain high fructose corn syrup?

Unfortunately, high fructose corn syrup has crept into so many foods it has become more and more difficult to avoid. Next time you go to the supermarket, read the nutritional labels. You will find high fructose corn syrup in common food items, such as soda, fruit like drinks, jam and syrup, frozen food, fruit canned in syrup, bread, fruit flavored yogurt, popsicles and ice pops, ketchup and BBQ sauce, salad dressing, jarred and canned pasta sauce, breakfast cereal, packaged dessert, and much more.

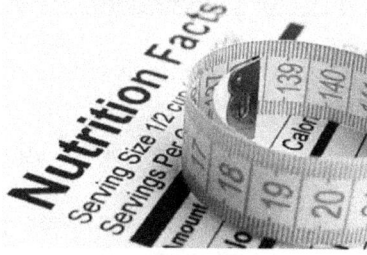

I know you may be saying, "Wow, that's nearly all of the things I shop for and feed my family when I go to the market! What's left to eat?"

Well, the key thing to remember is to feed your family the best foods possible that won't manifest sickness and disease in their bodies and will give them a longer better quality of life. Some of these foods you can still enjoy by preparing them naturally. Get your salad from *your* garden. Eat granola, dates, raisins, nuts, and oats for breakfast. Make ice cream or popsicles with natural fruit. Create your own sauces from home grown tomatoes, herbs, and other vegetables. Make your own jams and jellies. These are proactive ways to reduce and eliminate you and your family's consumption of high fructose corn syrup.

How can I avoid foods with high fructose corn syrup?

- ✓ Choose fresh whole produce (fruit & vegetables)
- ✓ Read the ingredients on food labels
- ✓ Limit processed foods and foods that contain sugar additives
- ✓ Avoid soda and processed fruit like drinks
- ✓ Drink water, fresh brewed tea, and squeezed juices
- ✓ Snack on whole foods such as various nuts and raw vegetables
- ✓ Bake sweet foods rather than store bought cakes, donuts, and cookies

Be cautious of the word *artificial* displayed on some food packaging. We never want to intentionally harm our bodies and our way of life.

11
Misconceptions

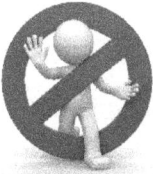

Let's dive deep and consider two questions to discover how we formed our views about food.

How did we begin to even learn about food?

What is the reason we eat certain things?

As children, our parents or another primary caregiver, introduced food to us. If we were not breastfed as a baby, we drank a form of milk (formula) mixed with water until the time came to introduce solid foods, such as cereal, fruits, and vegetables, and eventually meats and breads, right? Most of us have been encouraged to *eat* with clichés like, "Eat this, it will make you big and strong," and, "No dessert (or anything fun) until you finish your dinner." Usually when you hear a statement like that from someone, it is a badgering attempt to try to get you to eat something that looked or tasted unpleasant. This type of introduction to food did not really explore the content or nutritional value of what was to be consumed.

I don't know about you, but I didn't learn about the food pyramid until I entered school. The food groups and ideal number of daily servings were all illustrated in the form of a pyramid, displayed, and systematically taught. According to the food pyramid, a balanced diet equated to lots of bread, fruits and vegetables, some dairy, meats and proteins, and sparse consumption of fat, oil, and sweets.

Milk was presented as ideal for the human body, although it comes from a cow and is meant to feed the calf, not humans. Milk can contribute to intestinal problems and different types of meats knowingly contain antibiotics never meant for human consumption. Cheese, a milk product, can clog the intestines and raise cholesterol. Bread breaks down into sugar. Based on the research I have done; it seems as if there are several things wrong with the traditional food pyramid.

The nutritional importance of food was never explained to me until I developed diabetes as an adult. By way of a diabetes diagnosis, I found out pastas and breads breakdown into sugar. I think if I had learned about the nutritional value of food as a child, my eating habits would have been different. Life taught me, "It is going to make me big and strong," was not actually true. Most people grew up in households who expressed their culture and celebrated traditions with different types of foods. Certain holidays, birthdays, and other family gatherings come with foods that are not so good for our health. I will be the first to say, I definitely participated in the festivities without a second thought. I couldn't wait for get-togethers, so I could indulge. The fact of the matter is, I really didn't see the connection between food and my health, until I was diagnosed with diabetes, lupus, and fibromyalgia. It was not until then that I actually took the time to learn the nutritional value of the food I was eating and facts about how processed sugar, high fructose corn syrup, milk, and bread and other starches, had affected my health and my way of life. When I became conscious that *food is medicine*, and I could change my whole diagnosis, I was led to heal myself naturally and even raise my own food. The undisputable restoration of my health propels me to educate my children, grandchildren, and whoever is willing to listen or read this book to do the same.

I aim for my newfound love of agriculture to be contagious, inspire others to grow their own food, become more self-sufficient, and put their quality of life into their own hands.

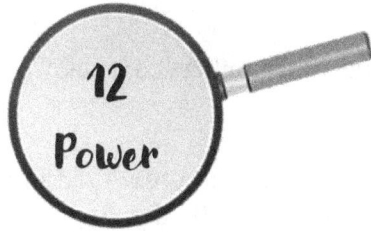

Self-sufficient (adj.): able to maintain oneself or itself without outside aid: capable of providing for one's own needs[1]

Independence (n.): the quality or state of being independent[2]

Independent (adj.): not requiring or relying on something else: not contingent[3]

Society subtly programs people to be dependent on outside forces, other than the sweat from their own brow. Many Americans have become slaves to the convenience of processed foods, contrary to what is ideal for their health and quality of life. Please, do not exchange your health for convenience.

One may argue, "There's not *that* much time in a day," because we have overfilled our lives with busyness. In the past, it was common for most people to grow their own food and the world was dependent on farmers and the natural way of things. My rebuttal, which I have shown evidence of in this book, is synthetic medications and their side effects, processed foods, and a poor diet keep people sick and diseased, robbing them of the time they value.

I am aware everyone is not capable nor doesn't have the land to grow their own food or raise their own animals for food. Alternatives are to shop at farmers' markets, whole food stores, and other outlets to obtain good quality fruits and vegetables.

There are also ways to grow food in limited space, without the use of harmful pesticides. Food can be planted in buckets or pots on balconies or porches if you live in an apartment, even inside, close to the window, if outside space is not available. These days, we have so much innovation. Food to supply you and your family can be grown using a hydroponic system, without the use of dirt. Many options are available to purchase or create tower gardens, inside or outside, to produce good quality natural grown food. The choice is yours. Yet again, it comes down to the quality of life you want, what you are willing to do, and the level of sacrifice you are willing to make to eliminate toxins, chemicals, processed sugars, and pesticides from your diet.

How can I become more self-sufficient?

- ✓ Start a garden
- ✓ Raise animals for food and / or income
- ✓ Compost to help the environment and reduce waste
- ✓ Recycle seeds
- ✓ Obtain a generator
- ✓ Store water, food, and supplies for future use

Water:

Be conscious of your ability to sustain yourself if there was a natural disaster, long-term power outage, drought, or food shortage. We must think about our future and prepare for the world to come. As the world stands today, self-sufficiency must be a priority. If we are honest, contaminates have been entering our water and food supply for years, in various forms:

> The per-and polyfluoroalkyl substances (PFAS) are a group of chemicals used to make fluoropolymer coatings and products that resist heat, oil, stains, grease, and water. Fluoropolymer coatings can be in a variety of products. These include clothing, furniture, adhesives, food packaging, heat-resistant non-stick cooking surfaces, and the insulation of electrical wire. Many PFAS, including perfluoro-octane sulfonic acid (PFOS) and perfluorooctanoic acid (PFOA), are a concern because they:
>
> - do not break down in the environment,
> - can move through soils and contaminate drinking water sources,
> - build up (bioaccumulate) in fish and wildlife.
>
> PFAS are found in rivers and lakes and in many types of animals on land and in the water.[4]

PFAS are a class of thousands of different chemicals. They are everywhere and turn up in everything from household items to fast food wrappers, to personal care products and cosmetics. They are even now prevalent in tap water.

> "USGS scientists tested water collected directly from people's kitchen sinks across the nation, providing the most comprehensive study to date on PFAS in tap water from both private wells and public supplies," said USGS research hydrologist Kelly Smalling, the study's lead author. "The study estimates that at least one type of PFAS – of those that were monitored – could be present in nearly half of the tap water in the

U.S. Furthermore, PFAS concentrations were similar between public supplies and private wells."[5]

Long story short, a lot of tap water isn't completely safe. As a part of becoming more self-sufficient and to protect our family, it is important to have a filtration system for our water. Also, store up water for natural disasters such as floods, hurricanes, and sewage system backups. These factors affect the water supply.

There are several different filtration systems on the market that are very affordable. Some fit on the kitchen faucet and shower nozzle. Larger, more costly units are available, but not necessary. Filtrated water can be stored in barrels or jugs for future use. I suggest each household maintain at least a 30-day supply of filtrated water in case something catastrophic happens. Tainted water is problematic. Preparation is a necessary component of self-sustainability.

Gardens:

Gardens are extremely valuable in many ways. Two ways to ensure your garden is well watered without becoming contaminated are to collect and store rainwater in barrels for future use and / or put a filtration system on your water hose.

The beautiful thing about starting a garden and learning about agriculture is the firsthand knowledge gained. Knowing how the food was grown, where it has been, and what you're consuming versus *not* knowing and taking a gamble.

There are many options to consider when planning your garden. When selecting what foods to grow, take note of the amount of space you have available, weather, season, water needs, and the time and resources it will take to keep the garden viable.

Ground Garden

Plant your food in a designated location directly 'in the ground'.

Raised Beds

Build a garden 'above' ground level (framed with wood, cinderblock, or use a ready to assemble kit). Then fill with soil.

Pots

Use various sized pots compatible with the food being grown. A benefit of using pots is they are more easily relocated when the weather changes.

Hydroponics

Eliminates soil and relies more heavily on nutrient filled water. Sizes of hydroponic systems range from small indoor designs to large outdoor options.

Aquaponics

Incorporates aquatic fish to naturally provide nutrients to the plants. This is another non-soil way to grow food.

Tower Gardens

A vertical design that allows multiple plants to be grown 'upwards' instead of over a surface area. Nutrient filled water is supplied to the plants through a hydroponic (water) or aeroponic (mist) system.

All these methods require tender love and care. You can't just put the seeds in the soil and forget about them. Tend to your food. If it's a ground crop, the garden area must be tilled, and the weeds pulled. The larger the area, the larger the harvest it will yield. If you build raised beds, be sure to clear fallen leaves, keep them watered, and fertilized. Even in pots, an abundance of food can be grown to sustain you and your family through a drought and / or winter.

All crops must be fertilized. Animals are an additional asset to becoming more self-sufficient because their waste acts as a great fertilizer.

Growing your own food is an achievable and rewarding task, on so many levels. It takes dedication and consistency and can be accomplished with little to no land.

Maximize your harvest. Plan ahead by storing up for winter or to help sustain your family through a food drought. Fresh fruits and vegetables can be purchased or bartered for from other farmers. As many as fifteen pounds of tomatoes can be supplied from just one self-watering patio container.

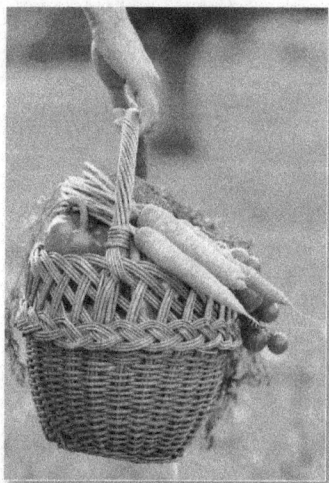

How do I decide what to grow?

Think about the things you and your family like to eat and begin there. Never plant food you don't eat and love. This way you'll have less waste.

How can I store the food I grow?

Preserve your harvest, which includes pickling, canning, drying, freezing, or possibly storing in a root cellar or underground coolant. Meat can also be persevered by canning, curing, raw packing, or hot packing.

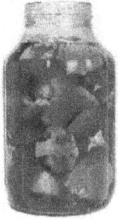

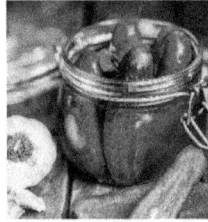

13
Homesteading

Deciding to become self-sufficient is definitely very rewarding. The most important thing to remember is that it is a choice. Deciding to take control of the way you live produces the life you desire and deserve for you and your family. Knowing what you're eating gives you control over what you are putting in your body and relinquishes that control from others. Choose to be healthy and not inadvertently contribute to sickness.

If you never *played* in the dirt, do not let that scare you away from the thought of growing even a flower. If there was no other way to feed your family or yourself, would you just starve or would you put your fingers in the dirt and grow something? "Better to be ready, so you don't have to get ready," my Auntie Diane would always tell me. Her words have forever stuck with me.

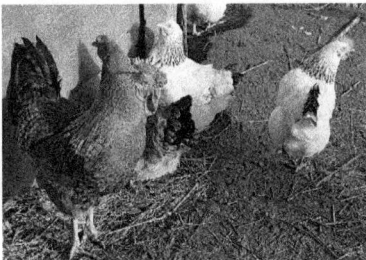

One way to achieve full self-sustainability is to venture out into homesteading. Once I made my mind up to truly make a commitment to raise something more than a dog, I had to figure out what type of animals would be suitable for my yard and the needs of my family. I knew I wanted chickens. I researched different types of chickens to determine which ones produced or laid the most eggs and had the best temperament. I have grandchildren so it was important to know which chickens were going to be friendly toward little children and which ones may try to attack.

Knowing I wanted the healthiest bird to start with, I chose to get quail. Quail are small fowl that don't require a lot of space and can be very easily kept in one- or two-tier cages or pens. The most important thing about quail is the nutritional value of their meat and eggs.

A single quail egg provides a significant chunk of daily Vitamin B12, selenium, riboflavin, and choline needs, along with some iron, all in a serving that contains only 14 calories.

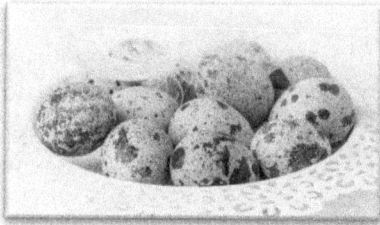

Selenium and riboflavin are important nutrients that help our body break down the food we eat and transform it into energy.

The next animals I decided to get were ducks. Duck eggs are also an excellent source of selenium, providing almost half of the recommended daily value in one egg.

Rabbits, also known as bunnies, are small mammals. They are great for a homestead because they can be raised in a small area. Their cages can be stacked on top of one

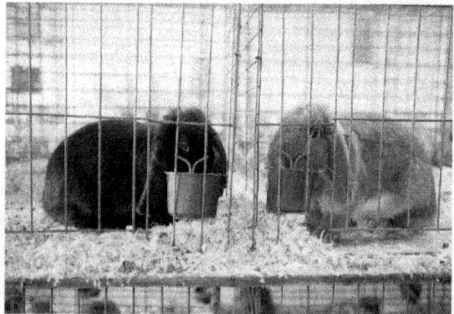

another. Rabbits' manure can be used for compost. It is organic and improves poor soil conditions, drainage, and moisture retention. These factors improve the life cycle of microorganisms in the soil. Worms love rabbit manure. It is not as smelly as other manures, is easily handled, and can be used right after it is expelled.

If you breed your rabbits, the babies can be sold to supply an income to help support your homestead. They are fast breeders and contribute to self-sufficiency.

The main focus of starting a homestead is to have better quality food to feed your body, with pure nutrients from animals you raised yourself, and are aware of what they're consuming because you are a part of the process. Home-steading is specific to *your* needs. Identify foods you and your family like to consume, or key components of your diet you could produce compatible with your homestead. Everyone isn't equipped to raise chickens, quail, ducks, or rabbits, but you can still become more proactive to improve your family's health. Plan for property or seek out local farmers markets that have grass chickens and other protein.

Homesteading is definitely *not* for the lazy. Animals are a consistent daily responsibility, and you genuinely have to be dedicated. They depend on you for everything, food and shelter. If they are not adequately tended to, health problems will arise. They also must be looked after if you leave your homestead for an extended period of time, or even just overnight. Scheduled feedings, watering, and habitat cleaning must be maintained as a part of a healthy living environment. Additional preparation and precautions must be made for changes in the weather.

Homesteading is obtainable and very rewarding for the health of you and your family. Growing your self-sustainability is a continual process. I would recommend taking one step at a time and moving forward little by little. It is hard work, but the aim is for it to be enjoyable and worthwhile, not overwhelming.

Herbs and garden structures were introduced in previous chapters. In this next section, we will go more into depth and grow in knowledge of gardening.

What should you put in my garden?

Most gardens consist of a mix of natural and constructed elements. Usually, some of the first things that come to mind are various florals, herbs, vegetables, shrubs, and trees, either intentionally planted or native, along with weeds. Many other creatures are also an interictal part of a garden's ecosystem, such as insects, arthropods, birds, soil, water, air, and sunlight.

When planning a garden, it is very important to think about what foods your family consumes. Please don't make the mistake of *just* planting anything or everything. If so, you'll have an abundance of food you don't have any need for. That overage will be a waste. Of course, if you have animals, you can use it for their food, but the purpose of the garden is to become more self-sufficient and supply your own source of nutrients for your family. Talk to your family and consider what preferred herbs, vegetables and fruits to include in your garden for seasoning, health benefits, teas, and to fulfill recipes. When planning my garden, I thought about the things that would be most beneficial for my household.

Here is a list of the ideal foods I grow in my garden (in alphabetical order) and some of their health benefits:

Aloe

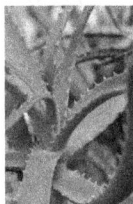

Contains healthy plant compounds that accelerate wound healing, reduce dental plaque, and help treat canker sores. Aloe helps reduce constipation and may improve skin appearance by preventing wrinkles. It also lowers blood sugar levels.

Beans

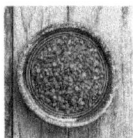

Contains plenty of fiber and protein. Boosts heart health. Good for diabetes control. Great source of iron. Provides magnesium and full of potassium.

Beets

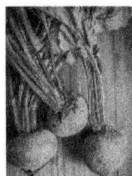

A plant root with many nutrients and few calories. May decrease elevated blood pressure, improve athletic performance, fight inflammation, improve digestive health, support brain health, and have anticancer properties.

Brussel Sprouts

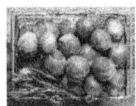

Protects against cancer of the stomach, lung, kidney, breast, bladder, and prostrate. Helps to ward off other health issues, such as high blood pressure, high cholesterol, heart disease, and diabetes.

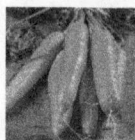

Carrots

Known to improve eye health. A good source of beta carotene, fiber, vitamin K1, potassium, and antioxidants. Lowers cholesterol levels, improves overall health, may provide anticancer effects, and assist with weight loss.

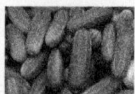

Cucumbers

Contains antioxidants, improves hydration, may aid in weight loss, lower blood sugar, and promote regularity. Easy to add to your diet.

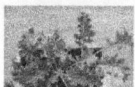

Kale

Rich in vitamin A (important for eye and bone health and promotes a strong immune system). Rich in vitamin C (combats colds and aids chronic disease prevention). Ideal source of vitamin K (helps blood clot and builds bones).

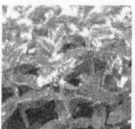

Oregano

Contains chemicals that may help reduce cough, aid digestion, and can fight against some bacteria and viruses. Oregano is used for wound healing, treating parasite infections, and many other conditions.

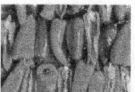

Peppers

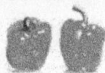

Rich in antioxidants associated with both better health and protection against conditions like heart disease and cancer. Packed with vitamin C and beta carotene.

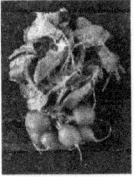

Radishes
Rich in antioxidants and minerals like calcium and potassium. Lowers high blood pressure and reduces risk of heart disease. Improves blood flow.

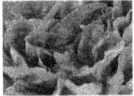

Romaine Lettuce
Low in fiber but high in minerals such as calcium, phosphorus, magnesium, and potassium. Naturally low in sodium and packed with vitamin C, vitamin K, and folate.

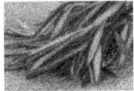

Rosemary
A rich source of antioxidants and anti-inflammatory compounds which are thought to help boost the immune system and improve blood circulation. Rosemary can also help to improve memory performance and quality, boosting alertness and focus.

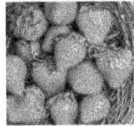

Strawberries
Rich in vitamin C and other antioxidants which help reduce the risk of serious health conditions like cancer, diabetes, stroke, and heart disease. Also, an excellent source of magnesium phosphorus.

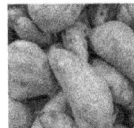

Sweet Potatoes
High in fiber and antioxidants which protect your body from damage caused by free radicals and promotes a healthy gut and brain.

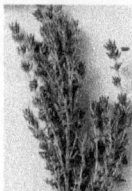

Thyme

Helps the body resist harmful organisms, supports respiratory health, promotes heart health, acts as a mood booster, encourages healthy looking skin, can be a natural bug repellent, is a powerful antioxidant, and soothes an occasional cough and sore throat.

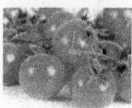

Tomatoes

Low in calories, provide important nutrients like vitamin C and potassium. Help reduce the risk of heart disease and certain cancers.

I truly believe *food is medicine*. Growing vegetables, herbs, and fruits on your homestead will add tremendous nutritional value to your diet and help *take your health into your own hands*. Committing to a better more self-sufficient way of life will ensure less chemicals, processed sugars, antibiotics, and plastics enter our bodies through food. We must consciously choose our future and the future of our family.

14
Be
Prepared

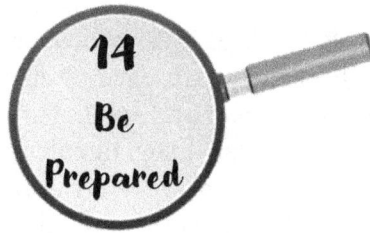

The world we live in today is becoming more and more polluted, corrupt, and systematic to the point where there is little to no concern for human life and the well-being of our planet. We must become proactive to lead and guide the upcoming generations back to healing the body naturally and becoming more self-sufficient.

We can't eliminate all water, soil, and air pollution on our own, but we can reduce its direct effect on us through our response to the knowledge we have. Begin filtrating your water. Use trusted soil for your garden and water it with filtered water or stored rainwater. You can also grow your food in a more controlled structure. There's not a lot we can do about all the chemicals entering the atmosphere (our air), except be aware and avoid contributing to the problem. We can reduce the negative impacts of any type of pollution by purposefully building up our immune system and keeping potassium iodine on hand for chemical warfare and / or sea moss that has natural iodine in it.

Natural Disaster Preparation

This is one of the chapters we definitely think we don't need, however, looking back over the years, it seems as if natural disasters are more frequent. Just think of the hurricanes and earthquakes around the world you have heard about showing up in places they were not expected, or peculiar times of the year considered 'out of season'. These natural disasters and other factors, such as overloaded or failing power grids, contribute to outages. Absence of electricity can contribute to contaminated water and food. Threats of war are on the rise, as well. All these things threaten the livelihood of your family and mine. Often, we don't want to admit these things are happening in the world around us, but the fact of the matter is they are.

We do not want another experience of panic and chaos like we did when the whole country was shut down during the Coronavirus (COVID) pandemic in 2020. People were scrambling for toilet paper and taking all the resources off the store shelves, inconsiderate of others. Learning from this, let us be prepared. Make sure your family is secure no matter what happens. Stock up on canned goods, water, first aid necessities, a generator, nonperishable foods like rice and beans, and store them in food safe containers. Take into consideration prescription and emergency medication supplies.

Be Prepared to Evacuate

Natural disasters arise quickly and may result in the need to evacuate. Sudden invasions of war may seem to be a thing of the past, but in this world we live in, we must be prepared. *Are you prepared to leave your home suddenly?* I recommend having a 'bug out bag' set aside with extra copies of identifying documents, titles / deeds, insurance, a first aid kit, tent, nonperishable foods, water, and other survival things. Make sure your family will be able to survive, even without electricity or shelter, for several days. Remember my Aunt Diane's words, "Be ready to keep from getting ready!"

Research ideal items for a bug out bag and decide which ones best meet the needs of your family. Here are some ideas:

Bug Out Bag Essentials
* ❖ Tarp or tent (emergency shelter)
* ❖ Paper map or compass
* ❖ Water
* ❖ High energy foods (lightweight to carry)
* ❖ Extra socks
* ❖ Multi-purpose tools
* ❖ Magnesium fire starter
* ❖ Hand cranked radio
* ❖ Sleeping bag(s)
* ❖ Clean clothes
* ❖ Cast iron pot (small enough to fit the bag)
* ❖ Important identification documents

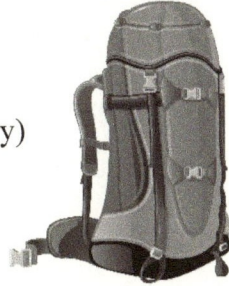

Survival Preparation

Being prepared is essential to your survival and your family's survival. We have to pay attention to the world we live in and not be ignorant of the enemy's devices. Please don't turn a blind eye to what's going on.

Here are some tips to assure you and your family are ready for whatever may happen in this world:

> **Water Contamination** – Ensure there is one gallon of water per person per day for several days, for drinking and sanitation. Depending on where you live, you can store water in large water barrels. Also keep water purification tablets on hand. They eliminate most bacteria and viruses from water by the gallons. This water can be used and / or stored for the future.

Food Storage – Have enough food stored for your family and yourself in case of a natural disaster, power grid shut down, and / or war. Nonperishable food items include dry goods and canned goods. Preserved foods can be stored in mason jars in a pantry or dark place. Beans, rice, and grains can be stored in food grade barrels and containers.

Make sure you have these items stored in your home as well:

1. A fire starter
2. Cast-iron pots and pans
3. Grill (charcoal or propane)
4. Tent
5. Batteries
6. Flashlights
7. Firearms for protection
8. Nonperishable foods
9. A generator
10. Paper map / compass
11. Battery powered or hand crank radio / NOAA weather radio with tone alert
12. Potassium iodine

Also, sit down with your family and make a survival plan. Include a contact procedure if there was a loss of modern communication, i.e. no telephone nor cell phone nor internet.

You may ask, "Why do I need *any* of this information?" Look around, this world is producing signs of the end times. Please be aware and prepare. Knowledge is power. Resources will be limited if everyone scrambles to make provisions at the same time.

Closing Prayer

People are sicker than they've ever been due to a lack of knowledge. I pray this book has enriched and blessed you. As we get back to the basics of things, know God has already blessed us indeed.

> Blessed be the God and Father of our Lord Jesus Christ, who has blessed us with every spiritual blessing in the heavenly places in Christ,
> -Ephesians 1:3

> For out of His fullness [the superabundance of His grace and truth] we have all received grace upon grace [spiritual blessing upon spiritual blessing, favor upon favor, and gift heaped upon gift].
> -John 1:16 AMP

I pray everything you have learned through reading this book enhances your life. Little by little, make the changes I advocate for. I believe with you for healing of your mind, body, and spirit. God did it for me, and I know He can do it for you too. Draw closer to our creator, Father God as He intended in the beginning.

Be aware of the way the world is turning - changes in our environment, the uncertainty of our water supply, abrupt power outages resulting from electrical overloads and natural disasters, and the uncertainty of war. Allow God to guide your preparations based on the needs of your family and the area where you live. God promises never to leave nor forsake us.

> And my God will liberally supply (fill until full) your every need according to His riches in glory in Christ Jesus.
> -Philippians 4:19 AMP

The Bible also teaches us, not to be ignorant of Satan's devices.

> [L]est Satan should take advantage of us; for we are not ignorant of his devices.
>
> -2 Corinthians 2:11

So, let's not perish because of a lack of knowledge.

> My people are destroyed for lack of knowledge [of My law, where I reveal My will].
>
> -Hosea 4:6 AMP

I pray that this book brings you knowledge, in the Name of Yeshua. Let's *Get Back to the Basics* together. Thank you for your support. Be blessed!

About the Author

Alia Wash is a wife, mother, grandmother, peer specialist, author, recovery advocate, and a self-taught herbalist. She was born in Newark, NJ in 1977 and was raised by her grandmother, from the age of three years old, in Cocoa, FL. She remembers, as a young child, spending time with her grandmother tending to her garden. At the time, she didn't realize how those years with Grandma created such a great impact in her life. Alia fondly remembers those foundational days when they lived a more self-sufficient life. Most of their diet was vegetables from the garden and wildlife her grandmother captured.

Later on in years, Alia's grandmother was diagnosed with breast cancer and given six months to live. She chose to use all natural remedies, without the help of doctors, and lived an additional fifteen years, far exceeding the given prognosis. This remarkable testimony was embedded in Alia's mind for most of her childhood into her adult life.

Alia was plagued with different types of diseases. After fifteen years of suffering from lupus, fibromyalgia, diabetes, and mental illness Alia put into practice the experiences she had with her grandmother throughout her childhood. She remembered the things her grandmother had taught her and how she lived longer than the doctor had predicted. Embarking upon her own journey, Alia was able to heal herself from lupus, fibromyalgia, diabetes, and mental illness. She no longer takes medication for these illnesses and has begun to help others heal themselves through natural medicine.

Alia continues her grandmother's legacy of hard work, research, and faith as she diligently pursues her own personal journey of health and agriculture to become more self-sufficient and heal herself naturally. It is her mission to reach back and help others learn how to do the same. But most importantly, to help the children of our future.

In pursuit of continued knowledge, excellence, and a strong desire to help others, Alia enrolled at Abraham Baldwin Agricultural College, in Georgia, to earn her bachelor's degree of agriculture in 2023. Never stop growing!

Learn more at: https://heavenscurenaturalfoods.com/

Or Email - Homesteading with the Washes:
aliawash6@gmail.com

Subscribe to *Homesteading with the Washes* on YouTube for more heathy lifestyle tutorial videos.

Additional Works

Learn more about Alia's story in her first book titled, *Why Not Recover*, 2018. *Why Not Recover*, is a tool designed to assist those who desire to relieve themselves from the bondage of addiction and the cycle of relapse. In this book you will receive the keys to obtain and maintain your freedom. Available on Amazon.com.

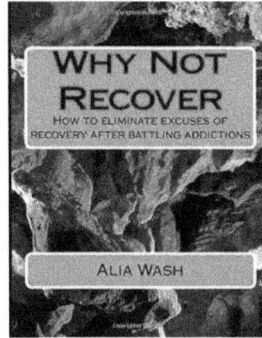

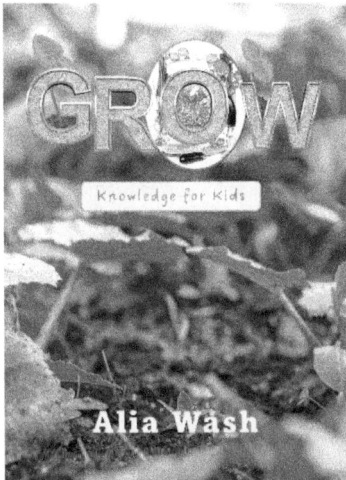

Alia's children's book, *Grow*, was released in 2023 and is ideal for the entire family! Available on Amazon.com.

Plant a seed in a child to learn about agriculture, nutrition, care for creation, and develop a love for the Creator.

Learn self-sustainability and the concept of food as medicine, through this engaging story of a grandmother lovingly reaching back and pouring knowledge into her grandson during a Spring Break of *'Homesteading with Grandma'* to remember.

Celebrate the generational love of family and the inspiration of wisdom for growth in children and adults alike.

End Notes

Chapter 1: Knowledge

[1] "Knowledge." Merriam-Webster.com Dictionary, Merriam-Webster, https://www.merr iamwebster.com/dictionary/knowledge. Accessed 31 Aug. 2023.

Chapter 3: Our Bodies

[1] Dr. William Li, *Masterclass with Dr. Li*, https://www.youtube.com/ watch?v=A2AClX qx2pY, (retrieved 9/15/23)

Chapter 4: Health-CARE

[1] Better Health Channel, https://www.betterhealth.vic.gov.au/health/healthyliving/water-a-vital-nutrient (retrieved 8/4/23)

[2] WebMD, WebMD Editorial Contributors, https://www.webmd.com/diabetes/what-is-ketosis (retrieved 8/5/23)

[3] Clevland Clinic, Autophagy, https://my.clevelandclinic.org/health/articles/24058-autop hagy#:~:text=Autophagy%20(pronounced%20%E2%80%9Cah%2DTAH,become%20de fective%20or%20stop%20working, (retrieved 8/8/23)

Chapter 5: Cell-CARE

[1] Healthline, *How many cells are in the human body? Fast Facts*, https://www. healthline.com/health/number-of-cells-in-body#:~:text=Most%20recent%20 estimates% 20put%20the,necessary%20for%20humans%20to%20survive.(retrieved 9/15/23)

[2] Medline Plus, National Library of Medicine, https://medlineplus.gov/ency/article/001 181. htm#:~:text=Acidosis%20is%20a%20condition%20in,base%20in%20the%20body %20fluids), retrieved 8/7/23.

[3] Canadian Cancer Society, *The Lymphatic System*, https://cancer.ca/en/cancer-information/what-is-cancer/lymphatic-system, retrieved 8/7/23.

[4] Dr. Axe, *Wormwood: The Parasite-Killing, Cancer-Fighting Super Herb* https://draxe. com/nutrition/wormwood/ (retrieved 8/20/23)

[5] RxList, *Wormwood*, https://www.rxlist.com/wormwood/supplements.htm (retrieved 8/20/23)

Chapter 7: Parasites

[1] Wikipedia contributors. "Parasitism." Wikipedia, The Free Encyclopedia. Wikipedia, The Free Encyclopedia, 1 Aug. 2023. Web.

[2] California Center for Functional Medicine, "What You Need to Know About Parasites", https://www.ccfmed.com/blog/parasites, (retrieved 8/10/23)

[3] Goldmann DA, Wilson CM. Pinworm infestations. In: Hoekelman RA. Primary pediatric care. 3d ed. St. Louis: Mosby, 1997:1519.

Chapter 8: Nutrition

[1] Piedmont, *Alkaline Diet*, https://www.piedmont.org/living-better/is-an-alkaline-diet-best-for-your-health#:~:text=Some%20background%3A%20The%20alkaline%20diet,

to%2201%20is%20considered%20alkaline. (retrieved 8/25/23)
[2] Waugh A, Grant A. *Anatomy and Physiology in Health and Illness. 10th edition.*
Philadelphia, Pa, USA: Churchill Livingstone Elsevier; 2007.

Chapter 10: Choices

[1] U.S. Food and Drug Administration, *High Fructose Corn Syrup Questions and Answers,*
https://www.fda.gov/food/food-additives-petitions/high-fructose-corn-syrup-questions-
and-answers (retrieved 8/31/23).
[2] Hartford Healthcare Hartford Hospital, *What Makes High Fructose Corn Syrup So Bad?*
https://www.hartfordhospital.org/about-hh/news-center/news-detail?articleId=27851&pu
blicid=461#:~:text=Weight%20gain%20abetted%20by%20high,visceral%20fat%20arou
nd%20your%20organs. (retrieved 8/31/23)

Chapter 12: Power

[1] "Self-sufficient." Merriam-Webster.com Dictionary, Merriam-Webster, https://www.me
rriam-webster.com/dictionary/self-sufficient. Accessed 31 Aug. 2023.
[2] "Independence." Merriam-Webster.com Dictionary, Merriam-Webster, https://www.mer
riam -webster.com/dictionary/independence. Accessed 31 Aug. 2023.
[3] "Independent." Merriam-Webster.com Dictionary, Merriam-Webster, https://www.mer
riam -webster.com/dictionary/independent. Accessed 31 Aug. 2023.
[4] Centers for Disease Control and Prevention, *Per- and Polyfluorinated Substances
(PFAS) Factsheet,* https://www.cdc.gov/biomonitoring/PFAS_FactSheet.html#:~:text=T
he%20per%2Dand%20polyfluoroalkyl%20substances,in%20a%20variety%20of%20prod
ucts. (Retrieved 9/1/23)
[5] USGS, *Tap water detects PFSA 'forever chemicals' across the US,* by Communications
Publishing, https://www.usgs.gov/news/national-news-release/tap-water-study-detects-
pfas-forever-chemicals-across-us#:~:text=USGS%20estimates%20at%20least
%2045,have%20one%20or%20more%20PFAS&text=At%20least%2045%25%20of%20t
he,by%20the%20U.S.%20Geological%20Survey. (Retrieved 9/1/23)